# Body Building

Proven Bodybuilding Techniques For Effective Muscle, Strength And Mass Building Within A 30-day Timeframe

*(Comprehensive Guide: Nutritional And Supplement Strategies For Male Bodybuilders)*

## Piotr Baker

# TABLE OF CONTENT

# Introduction

If your ambition is to efficiently increase your muscle mass within a shorter timeframe, then you have arrived at the appropriate destination. This book has been specifically crafted for individuals who desire to acquire muscle mass efficiently and minimize any time spent in doing so. We expeditiously commence our focus on the matter, promptly addressing all significant facets of muscular development in a comprehensive manner. We shall engage in a comprehensive conversation regarding appropriate dietary practices, physical exercises, and nutritional supplements that can aid in the attainment of your desired physique.

Undoubtedly, achieving the desired outcome will require a considerable amount of time and diligent dedication. However, by faithfully adhering to the guidance provided in this book, success is assuredly within reach. Drawing from my personal expertise, I have utilized the wealth of knowledge gained from reflecting upon the errors I committed during my endeavors. By perusing this book, you can bypass the pitfalls that stemmed from those identical mistakes.

The purpose of this book is to provide comprehensive guidance and encompass all necessary knowledge to efficiently and expeditiously achieve a well-toned physique.

Session three
This session focuses primarily on the lower extremities and lumbar region.

Standing squats
This exercise targets the muscles of the upper thighs. Additionally, it effectively targets the gluteal and lumbar muscles.

Use a squat rack. Don\\\'t use a machine. A machine inhibits locomotion and hinders the body's ability to follow its innate trajectory. Consequently, your muscular growth will be hindered.

Commence by placing the barbell in the squat rack, ensuring that it is properly supported. If you commence with the weight positioned on the ground, you may encounter difficulty in raising it to the level of your shoulders for proper handling.

The optimal height is at the same level as the upper portion of your chest. This will enable you to maintain contact between your feet and the floor while raising the weight from the rack.

Assuming a position in front of the bar, proceed to move beneath it in such a manner that the load rests upon the upper region of your shoulders. Please ensure that it is positioned below your neck. The application of excessive weight upon your neck is likely to result in physical harm.

Maintain a stance with your feet positioned at shoulder width, oriented slightly outward.

Grasp the bar, maintaining a distance between your hands equal to the width of your shoulders. This will help maintain a firm posture, ensuring that the load is properly distributed along the spine. Employ an overhand grip, ensuring that the thumbs are positioned atop. Ensure that the weight remains securely positioned against the posterior region of your upper shoulder.

Once prepared, please step back by two paces. This is at a distance of approximately four to six feet from the rack.

Please maintain a forward gaze, align your spine in a straight position, and extend your chest outward. Do not look up. Engaging in such behavior may lead to potential harm to the neck region. Maintain a forward gaze throughout the entirety of the motion. This measure will guarantee accurate alignment and prevent any potential harm.

Ensure that the barbell maintains a vertical trajectory throughout the entirety of the exercise. Strive to maintain alignment of the barbell with the midpoint of your feet as you execute the upward and downward motions. In addition, ensure that your knees do not extend past your toes. Maintain proper posture by ensuring that your back remains erect and your chest is prominently extended forward.

Ensure that your hips are positioned slightly lower than your knees at the lowermost point. Ensure that the knees are positioned in a slightly outward direction directly above the feet. Maintain proper postural alignment by ensuring a straightened back while angling the body forward at an approximate angle of 45 degrees. This will guarantee that the weight is maintained above the midpoint of your feet. Starting from this stance, ascend while ensuring that the barbell remains centered directly above the midpoint of your feet.

It would be advisable to initially engage in the motion without incorporating any additional weight. By following this approach, you will guarantee the correctness of your actions.

Dead lift
Commence by placing the bar in a horizontal position on the ground. Please position your feet in a stance that is slightly narrower than shoulder width, ensuring that your toes are pointing slightly outward. Ensure that the bar is aligned precisely above the midpoint of your feet. Maintain this specific position consistently throughout the entirety of the exercise.

Securely grasp the bar while ensuring that both palms are oriented in a reverse direction. Ensuring a secure grip, encircle the bar with your thumbs to prevent any slipping. Adopt a grip on the bar that is equivalent to the width of your shoulders.

Elevate the bar by ascending in a vertical fashion. Maintain an upright posture by aligning the spine, protruding the chest, and maintaining forward-facing gaze throughout the entirety of the exercise. Do not engage in excessive back arching as it may increase the risk of injury. Employ the complete extent of motion, encompassing the downward trajectory until contact with the floor is made, subsequently ascending back up in its entirety.

Calve raises
This exercise effectively engages the entire set of muscles in the calf region.

Maintain a firm grip on the barbell while fully extending your arms. Assume a position on a platform of approximately three inches in height. Position the anterior portion of your feet on the block, while maintaining the remainder of your feet elevated above the floor.

Maintaining an erect posture, elevate and descend your physique by executing flexion movements with your feet. Ensure you achieve a substantial stretch at the nadir of the motion.

Execute six repetitions in each set.

During this session, you have engaged and exercised your leg and lower back muscles.

## Abdominals and buttocks

It is recommended that these exercises are performed at the conclusion of each session. Resist the temptation to engage in these activities with increased frequency. All that will be achieved is an excessive stimulation of the muscles, leading to potential overtraining.

### Abdominal crunches
This exercise targets and engages the entirety of the abdominal region.

Assume a prone position on the floor. Please ensure that you flex your knees and maintain contact between your feet and the floor.

Please position your hands on both sides of your head. Gradually elevate your physique towards your knees employing a rolling action. Namely, steadily shift your body forward, incrementally, commencing with your head.

In essence, you are executing a movement where your body is being propelled towards your knees. This is an audible movement. You are contracting the muscles in your abdomen.

Perform three sets of maximal repetitions.

Bicycle crunches
This exercise specifically focuses on the abdominal muscles situated laterally on both sides of the body.

This movement, similar to the aforementioned exercise, involves a repetitive and forceful contraction.

There exists a distinction in that one shoulder is rotated individually towards the knee on the opposite side.

Commence by assuming a prone position on the ground. Please flex your knees and maintain the soles of your feet in contact with the floor. Position your hands bilaterally alongside your head, ensuring that your elbows are directed forward.

Please rotate your left shoulder in the direction of your right knee. Extend your body to its full capacity and subsequently retract back to a supine position on the ground. Perform the same action utilizing your right shoulder.

Please perform as many iterations as possible.

Lying scissors spread
This exercise is highly effective for toning and sculpting the gluteal muscles. Additionally, it provides employment

opportunities for the muscles in your lower back.

Assume a prone position on the floor. Please position your hands beneath your hips.

Elevate both of your legs as much as possible, with the aim of lifting them off the floor. Continue without ceasing and proceed to extend your legs laterally. Realign the objects in their original position, and subsequently lower them back onto the floor. Continuing without interruption, elevate your legs in order to initiate another repetition.

Execute three sets comprising the maximum number of repetitions attainable.

The most straightforward and uncomplicated nutritious eating plan on a global scale.

Are you interested in adopting a nutritious and uncomplicated dietary regimen? Well, here it is.

Consume food at your discretion and in accordance with your body's nutritional requirements. Please heed the signals and cues your body provides. Use common sense. Avoid rubbish. Consume lean protein, fresh produce, and whole grains. That\\\'s your diet.

Numerous individuals encounter complexity in adhering to dietary plans. They engage in the practice of monitoring caloric intake, protein content, and carbohydrate levels. This is all unnecessary.

The human physique functions as an inherent mechanism for survival. It indicates the appropriate times for consumption and when satiety has been reached.

As you mature, your dietary requirements increase. Nevertheless, there is no requirement for you to exert deliberate intentionality. The metabolic demands of an individual tend to increase proportionally with their body size, resulting in a higher expenditure of calories. Hence, it will inherently indicate the appropriate moments to initiate and conclude your meals.

What about low fat? Consuming food sources that are rich in saturated fat has long been recognized to have adverse effects on one's overall well-being. Nevertheless, this is a fundamental principle that should be apparent to all. There is no requirement for you to compile a list of foods that are high in fat. Your rationality will guide you in determining what actions or choices to refrain from.

It remains a verifiable reality that the growth of your muscles can still occur when nourished with suboptimal dietary choices. Nevertheless, it is not solely a matter of nourishing your muscles.

It\\\'s also about health. Your well-being holds utmost significance.

Once more, exercise sound judgment. It is widely acknowledged that a well-balanced dietary regimen encompasses lean proteins, fresh produce, specifically fruits and vegetables, and whole grain products. Adhering to these food choices will lead to positive impacts on your overall well-being.

It is advisable to refrain from the use of chemicals. These are frequently employed by manufacturers in food products. Do not unnecessarily complicate matters for yourself. Merely peruse the roster of components.

When consuming fruits and vegetables, it is advisable to thoroughly wash them prior to consumption. This precaution is being taken in the event that the produce still retains traces of pesticides. These are frequently employed for the purpose of deterring insects. Ensure that these are removed by washing them before consumption.

All of these concepts can be easily understood through logical reasoning.

Consume vegetables, lean protein, and fresh produce. The following food items are considered to be nutritious and beneficial for one's health. They exhibit a low fat content and comprise all the essential nutrients required to sustain the body.

There is no need to be concerned with calorie counting. Your physique is naturally adapted to ensure survival. It will indicate the appropriate timings for meals. Consume food when you are aware of your nutritional requirements.

There is a plethora of research indicating that consuming frequent smaller meals is advantageous for one's well-being. This phenomenon occurs due to the inherent limitation of the human body to assimilate a finite quantity within any specific timeframe. When an excessive amount is ingested beyond the body's requirements, it will expel the excess. It will be either eliminated through excretion or stored as adipose tissue. Therefore, just eat enough. You will be able to ascertain when you have consumed an adequate amount. Your body will cease to experience sensations of hunger.

Section One: Establishing Your Nutritional Base

A bodybuilding diet may be formulated based on dietary components, as well as structured with consideration to the macro composition of nutrients, namely protein, carbohydrates, and fats. In order to accomplish this task proficiently, it is imperative for bodybuilders to have a comprehensive understanding of the precise quantities of carbohydrates, proteins, and fats that they are consuming on a daily basis.

The quantities, varieties, and proportions of macronutrients ingested (and their timing) are indicative of the overall sufficiency of a bodybuilding diet. Additional nutrients, such as water and fiber, play a vital role in the diet of bodybuilders and should also be taken into careful consideration.

Ensure an Adequate Protein Intake

It is our recommendation that individuals engaged in bodybuilding consume a minimum of one gram of protein per pound of body weight daily, and in the case of hardgainers, even up to nearly two grams per pound. The protein requirements for individual bodybuilders may fluctuate, however, adhering to this minimum threshold guarantees adequate quantities for the purpose of muscle growth.

In the event that your body weight is relatively low or if your caloric requirements for maintenance are elevated, it is possible that you might necessitate a greater protein intake compared to individuals of similar stature who are engaged in bodybuilding.

Consume an ample amount of carbohydrates to sustain energy levels.

The human body has the ability to utilize protein, carbohydrates, or fats as sources of energy. However, when engaging in intense physical training, the body tends to preferentially prioritize the utilization of carbohydrates. Consuming a sufficient amount of carbohydrates facilitates efficient energy production in the body, thereby preserving protein and fats for their respective specialized nutritional functions.

Emphasize Slow-Digesting Carbs

Complex carbohydrates are comprised of elongated chains of sugars. The majority, albeit not all, of complex carbohydrates exhibit a slow digestibility. Emphasize the consumption of whole-grain products (such as whole-wheat bread and pasta, oatmeal, brown rice, etc.), as well as sweet potatoes, as they have a slower digestion rate compared to white bread and white potatoes, along with sugars which have a faster digestion rate. Carbohydrates that are metabolized slowly offer sustained energy and are less likely to be stored as adipose tissue. During a phase dedicated to muscle growth, it is advisable to consume a minimum of 2 grams and up to approximately 3 grams of carbohydrates per pound of bodyweight per day. In the process of trimming phases, it is advisable to lower overall carbohydrate intake to 1 gram per pound of body weight.

De-Emphasize Simple Carbs

With the exception of post-workout periods, it is advisable for a bodybuilder to reduce their intake of calories derived from simple carbohydrates (sugar). Highly accessible, simple carbohydrates can undergo rapid absorption, particularly when consumed in liquids low in fats or devoid of solid foods, thus experiencing unhindered transit through the gastrointestinal tract. Substantial amounts of simple carbohydrates elicit the secretion of insulin, which is favorable in the post-exercise period but not during other times, as it may stimulate the body to store these sugars as adipose tissue. Foods that have a high sugar content are considered among the most detrimental for individuals engaged in bodybuilding who aim to maintain a low body fat percentage.

Minimize consumption of saturated fats while avoiding the consumption of trans fats.

The surplus of these two varieties of fat intensify the susceptibility to cardiac and other medical complications, while also compromising endeavors in physique development. Trans fats are frequently present in processed food items such as crackers, cookies, and other baked consumables. Saturated fats are abundant in cuts of meat that are of lower quality and have a higher fat content.

Consume Healthy Fats

Foods that are rich in unsaturated fats, especially monounsaturated fats, are highly beneficial for individuals who engage in bodybuilding. Do not subscribe to the belief that a bodybuilding diet must contain minimal fat – instead, it should strictly limit the intake of saturated and trans fats.

Omega-3 fatty acids, which can be derived from sources such as fish and flaxseed oils, play a crucial role in establishing an advantageous hormonal milieu to facilitate muscle tissue growth and promote leanness.

Additionally, unsaturated fats present in olives, avocados, nuts, seeds, as well as olive and canola oils, offer bodybuilders a plethora of muscle-building benefits. With the exception of reducing portions, fats should constitute 20%-30% of your daily dietary intake.

Count Calories

During the analysis of a bodybuilding diet, macronutrients are frequently divided into percentages. As an example, a dietary suggestion during the offseason could be to obtain 50% of total caloric intake from carbohydrates, 30% from protein, and 20% from fats. In order to ensure precision, it is imperative to possess this invaluable information: each gram of carbohydrates contains approximately four calories, each gram of protein carries four calories, and each gram of fat provides as much as nine calories. This disparity in caloric intake elucidates the rationale behind bodybuilders, including those who do not adhere to a low-fat dietary regimen, being required to conscientiously consider the consumption of fat calories in addition to carbohydrates and protein. Regarding the objective of increasing one's body mass, it is recommended to aim for a minimum of 20 calories per pound of body weight. To facilitate the process of achieving a lean physique, it is advisable to reduce calorie intake to a maximum of 15 calories per pound of body weight.

Consume a minimum of one gallon of water daily.

Water is indispensable for general well-being and plays a crucial role in muscle development. Maintaining adequate hydration of your body offers benefits ranging from the synthesis of protein to the process of digestion. Consistent water consumption facilitates the circulation of nutrients within your bloodstream, ensuring their transportation into muscle cells. Water is furthermore an indispensable provider of numerous essential minerals. However, it is advisable not to consume the entire gallon in a single session; instead, it is recommended to ingest it gradually throughout the course of the day. This holds particular significance for individuals engaging in bodybuilding regimens that involve high-protein diets, as well as those who incorporate substances like creatine, fat burners, or other supplementary compounds that exert an influence on the body's hydration status. Please bear in mind that water maintains the fullness of your muscles. Furthermore, scientific studies have demonstrated that consuming a mere two cups of water in the intervals between meals can aid in weight management by enhancing metabolic rate. Water is vital for sustaining life, and its significance to individuals engaged in bodybuilding cannot be overstated. Consume a pint of water during principal meals and endeavor to surpass the daily recommended intake of one gallon.

Fire Up Your Fiber

Many bodybuilding dietary choices are well-known for their relatively low fiber content; nevertheless, bodybuilders require a substantial intake of fiber to achieve optimal gains. Bodybuilders should obtain a significant portion of their dietary fiber from sources such as complex carbohydrates, fruits, and vegetables. Make an effort to consume a daily intake of 30 grams of dietary fiber, and increase this amount further when following a high-calorie dietary plan. If your diet fails to meet this requirement, it is advisable to contemplate daily supplementation using a fiber-based supplement.

Meat Makes Muscle

Various types of protein are beneficial for bodybuilders aiming to increase muscle mass, yet among the most optimal choices are lean varieties of meat. Turkey, chicken, beef, and other varieties of meat are rich in complete proteins, as they encompass all the essential amino acids required by the body. In contrast, alternative protein sources, particularly those derived from vegetables, are incomplete and therefore less concentrated in terms of protein content.

To achieve optimal outcomes, I suggest that bodybuilders endeavor to incorporate animal protein into their meals on a consistent basis. Some notable options for meat selection include chicken and turkey breast, as well as lean cuts of red meat.

Incorporate both fatty and low-fat fish into your diet.

Fish, being an exceptional protein source, ought to be regularly consumed by individuals engaged in bodybuilding endeavors. Fish can have varying levels of fat content, with certain types being rich in healthy fats while others contain little to no fat. However, in contrast to other tissue proteins, fatty fish offer a multitude of advantages to bodybuilders. Salmon and sardines, for instance, are noteworthy providers of omega-3 fatty acids, profoundly contributing to bolstering the immune system while aiding in the recuperation and development of muscles, among various other advantages, including facilitating fat loss. Fish that possess lesser fat content, such as tilapia, additionally serve as a commendable protein source. It is recommended that individuals engaged in bodybuilding endeavors, regardless of their specific dietary or training objectives, aim to consume a minimum of two servings, each consisting of eight ounces, of fatty fish per week.

Employing grains and starches in a suitable manner" "Utilizing grains and starches accordingly" "Incorporating grains and starches as deemed fitting" "Adopting an appropriate approach to the utilization of grains and starches

Certain bodybuilders tend to abstain from the consumption of grains such as brown rice and whole wheat products, predominantly due to their high carbohydrate content. Others incorporate generous amounts of pasta, cereal, and bread into their dietary patterns. As a rule, it is advisable to incorporate grains into your diet;

however, it is important to be mindful of their impact on your physical well-being. Certain bodybuilders are capable of consuming them daily with minimal impact. It is necessary for others to diligently observe the amount they consume. However, it is imperative that all individuals engaged in bodybuilding consciously choose whole-grain alternatives as opposed to processed grains.

Incorporate Vegetables into Your Daily Diet

Regrettably, vegetables often fail to receive adequate recognition as essential constituents of bodybuilding nutrition. Numerous bodybuilders demonstrate strict adherence to their protein and complex carbohydrate intake, yet tend to disregard consuming an adequate quantity and assortment of vegetables. Bodybuilders should aim to consume five or six servings on a daily basis. In order to cater to your requirements, it is advisable to incorporate multiple servings during a meal. Vegetables not only offer essential nutrients that may be deficient in other bodybuilding foods, but they also contribute to satiety and aid digestion due to their fibrous composition, thereby enhancing the effectiveness of a high-protein diet.

Fruit Offers Essential Nutrients and Dietary Fiber.

Several bodybuilders tend to overlook fruit, just as they neglect vegetables. Fruit serves as a highly beneficial source of dietary fiber, carbohydrates, antioxidants, and a multitude of additional essential nutrients. Majority of fruits constitute a source of carbohydrates that are digested at a slower rate.

Fruit also provides essential nutrients that are difficult to obtain from other sources of food for bodybuilding. Consume a variety of fruits, ensuring the intake of two or more pieces or servings per day. Fruits serve as an excellent source of carbohydrates for pre-workout fuel.

Section Two: Additional Guidelines

Supplements constitute an integral element of your bodybuilding nutritional strategy; however, they are merely one constituent. By keeping that in mind, one can gain a significant advantage through the utilization of supplementation.

Supplement Intelligently

Supplements serve as a means to facilitate the attainment of your objectives. They do not possess the enchanting properties to fulfill the desired form of your physique. It is imperative to employ supplements judiciously, while maintaining reasonable expectations of their potential benefits for oneself. You are still required to undergo training and adhere strictly to your specified dietary regimen. If you diligently engage in the laborious efforts and appropriately utilize the supplements as intended, you shall reap the desirable advantages that you aspire to derive from them.

Use Protein Supplements

Consume a protein supplement a minimum of once daily on days of rest and twice daily on days of physical exercise. Opting for a product manufactured by a reputable company will enable you to supplement your daily protein intake by an additional 40-80 grams. Moreover, this approach will assist in aligning with our accepted protein guideline, which advises consuming a minimum of 1 gram of protein for every pound of bodyweight on a daily basis. It is frequently sufficient to induce a substantial advancement in muscular development, typically discernible within a span of four months. It is particularly crucial to adhere to this formula when engaging in a dietary regimen. Given the elevated requirements for protein and the necessity to limit calorie consumption, a protein supplement becomes indispensable.

Consume approximately 20 grams of protein powder, such as whey, prior to commencing your workouts and around 40 grams immediately following your exercise sessions. During days of rest, it is advisable to ingest a protein shake weighing at least 40 g in between meals.

Utilize a Comprehensive Multivitamin Supplement

Consume a multivitamin during breakfast and dinner on a daily basis to ensure proper nourishment. A deficiency in any vitamin can result in disruptions to the foundation of muscle formation. The convergence of a fast-food society with the specific nutritional needs of bodybuilding can result in a deficiency in a multitude of essential micronutrients. It is unfortunate to note that a significant number of them are required for activities that pertain to an individual primarily focused on muscle building and fat reduction, which are of great interest to them.

Mix Your Antioxidants

Consume a combination of antioxidants; a well-balanced mixture exerts an anticatabolic impact by suppressing the formation of free radicals both during and subsequent to rigorous physical exertion. Please consider incorporating our recommended high-ranking choices into your antioxidant regimen: 400-800 IU of vitamin E, 500-1,000 mg of vitamin C, and 200 mcg of selenium. Obtain the remainder of your daily portions of fruits and vegetables.

Vitamin C Can Rejuvenate and Energize Your Body

Vitamin C serves as a potent antioxidant, facilitating the synthesis of hormones, amino acids, and collagen. In addition, it safeguards immune system cells from harm, thereby enhancing their effectiveness and productivity.

The human body lacks the ability to retain vitamin C, therefore it must be regularly supplemented. Although multivitamins include vitamin C, supplementary intake will guarantee the avoidance of any deficiency. Consume a daily dosage ranging from 1,000 to 2,000 mg.

Vitamin E is highly beneficial.

This particular antioxidant exhibits significant protective properties towards bodily tissues. Vitamin E functions as an antioxidant that safeguards a multitude of substances from detrimental degradation within the human body. Additionally, Vitamin E extends the lifespan of erythrocytes and is crucial for the adequate utilization of oxygen by the muscular system. It is advisable for bodybuilders to take a daily supplementation dose ranging from 400 to 1,200 IU. Consume 400 international units (IU) of vitamin E during breakfast, and another 400-800 IU alongside your post-workout shake.

# Procedures to Follow in Order to Develop Substantial Physical Power!

Outlined below are the fundamental procedures that you should adhere to in order to acquire substantial muscular strength capable of yielding impactful outcomes. Simply adhere to these three sequential actions, and you shall undoubtedly progress towards becoming an authentic exemplar of physical strength, regardless of gender.

Step 1: Implementing Progressive Overload:

This principle is fundamental within the compendium of constructing resilience. Progressive overload refers to the gradual increase in weight or resistance over time after initially starting with a manageable load, resulting in the ability to lift increasingly heavier weights. As an illustration, if an individual can successfully perform 5 repetitions of deadlift or squat with a maximum weight of 200 lbs, they should proceed by rehearsing with this weight. Sequentially, they may gradually increase the load by a small increment, such as 5 lbs, on a weekly basis. This will result in progressing the weight incrementally to 205 lbs, then gradually to 210 lbs, and so forth. You can observe the events unfolding here!

Step 2: Enhance Tension to the Maximum Level:

The key to developing strength lies in the application of tension. Strength can be described as the capacity of the musculature in the body to generate tension. Muscular tension is equivalent to force, and force is equivalent to tension. Enhance muscular exertion by regularly partaking in the lifting of heavier weights. If we are discussing bodyweight exercise and you possess exceptional proficiency in performing conventional push-ups, I would suggest substituting a set of 100 regular push-ups with 5 repetitions of one-arm push-ups. Reduced repetitions, yet increased tension! Through consistent application of this technique, one will gradually cultivate and enhance physical strength. This is the reason why powerlifters possess such formidable strength.

Step 3: Compound Exercises:

This is an unequivocal principle for the development of muscular prowess. To efficiently develop significant strength, it is advisable to avoid allocating excessive time to exercises such as isolated bicep curls. Rather than engaging in bicep curls, opt for performing pull-ups instead. Besides working the bicep muscles, the exercise engages the latissimus dorsi, trapezius, deltoids, and biceps. This is the factor that also arouses your autonomic nervous system and triggers your body's innate generation of growth hormone and testosterone. I encourage you to give it a try.

Strategies for Rapidly Developing Larger Arms - 4 Effective Exercises for Achieving Significant Arm Growth

Prominent, robust biceps serve as a key indicator of overall physical prowess. Posessing well-developed arms can significantly alter an individual's appearance and levels of self-assurance. Individuals consistently devote countless hours at the gym, diligently engaging in weightlifting exercises, with the ultimate objective of attaining substantial arm muscles. Regrettably, the somber reality remains that a significant portion of these individuals will never succeed in developing aesthetically pleasing arms due to their lack of familiarity with the essential requirements for achieving such muscularity.

The issue that many individuals encounter is that they allocate a significant portion of their attention towards the development of their biceps, despite the fact that, in actuality, the biceps constitute the smallest segment of one's arms.

To acquire knowledge regarding the key to developing substantial arms, it is imperative to possess a deep understanding of the anatomical structure of one's arms. The bicep muscle is situated superiorly on the upper arm and constitutes approximately one-third of the arm's overall composition. The triceps muscle is located on the distal region of the brachium and constitutes approximately two-thirds of the arm. Additionally, a region that merits attention is the group of muscles situated in the forearm, which are often overlooked despite comprising the entirety of the lower arm.

Presented herein are four supplementary exercises that can be incorporated alongside your bicep training regimen, thereby facilitating substantial growth of the upper arm musculature.

Tricep Extension

This particular tricep exercise holds a position of high regard in my repertoire, owing to its merit as a compound movement that effectively engages all three facets of the tricep muscle. To execute this exercise, assume a supine position on the ground while ensuring the barbell is positioned on the floor before your head.

Take hold of the bar slightly narrower than the width of your shoulders and raise it so that the bar is positioned above your chest. Subsequently, proceed to lower the weight using solely your lower arms, maintaining the position of the bar slightly above your head, while refraining from any movement of your upper arms. Maintain the position for a duration of one second before elevating the weight back to its initial pose.

Compact Hand Placement Bench Press

This particular exercise is a compound movement that effectively engages all three heads of the tricep. To execute this exercise, simply assume the set-up position usually employed for a conventional bench press. To deviate from grasping the bar with a width equal to or exceeding the distance between your shoulders, you will henceforth position your hands approximately 10 inches apart from each other.

It is crucial to acknowledge that maintaining low proximity between your elbows and your body is highly recommended, as it aids in concentrating the effort on your triceps rather than on your chest. Now, you simply execute the movements associated with a bench press.

## Wrist Flexion/ Wrist Extension

Now that we have addressed the upper arm, it is equally imperative that we attend to the lower arm. Nothing appears more preposterous than the incongruity of well-developed upper arms juxtaposed with underdeveloped forearms in an individual. To execute the wrist curls, simply assume a seated position on a bench or chair. Grasp the barbell and position your hands approximately 8 inches apart.

Extend your legs so that the upper part of your forearms rests on them, while permitting your wrists to naturally hang over your knees. Now, your task is to gradually decrease the weight and allow it to descend along your fingertips, subsequently curling it back up to its initial position.

The reverse wrist curls can be described as a similar exercise, albeit with a variation in hand positioning. Instead of grasping the weight from beneath with an underhand grip, it is grasped from above with an overhand grip. Moreover, instead of placing the tops of the forearms on the legs for support, the bottoms of the forearms are simply rested on the legs.

Strategies for Developing Significant Muscularity through Creatine Supplementation

The consumption of creatine has the potential to significantly enhance one's energy levels during physical exercise. There are numerous advantages that can be obtained by consuming this supplement:

Enhanced physical stamina during exercise owing to the restoration of ATP.

Enhanced muscular strength to perform more challenging exercises during your workout.

A reduction in the process of glycolysis results in a lower production of lactic acid.

Assist in facilitating rapid weight gain, taking into consideration your previous non-consumption of creatine.

ATP, known as Adenosine Triphosphate, serves as the primary energy source to facilitate muscle contraction. The liberation of a single phosphate from adenosine triphosphate (ATP) generates additional energy for the purpose of lifting weights. Through the consumption of creatine, you are providing your body with an increased supply of phosphate. Subsequently, this phosphate will undergo a reaction with ADP, resulting in the formation of ATP. The greater quantity of ATP available to you, the higher additional energy can be acquired during weightlifting.

The process of ATP regeneration serves to prevent the body from depending on glycolysis, a metabolic pathway that ultimately results in the production of lactic acid. This advantage is evident: reducing the production of lactic acid allows you to engage in more extensive and intense physical exercise. Each repetition performed during a workout session can be advantageous and yield benefits for you. You will acquire greater mass and strength. One additional advantage associated with the consumption of creatine is its ability to prevent fatigue during weightlifting.

The notion that creatine lacks benefits is unfounded. Substantial increases in muscle mass can be achieved within a brief timeframe, particularly among individuals who have previously not incorporated creatine supplementation into their regimen. It demonstrates enhanced efficacy when combined with whey protein. Throughout the process of recuperation, it is imperative to adequately provide your body with sufficient protein to effectively restore and mend your muscles. Proteins undergo enzymatic decomposition, resulting in the formation of amino acids, which serve as the fundamental constituents for the development and maintenance of muscle tissues.

Individuals who struggle to build muscle mass can effectively enhance their gains through the utilization of creatine. The typical increase generally amounts to a range of ten to twenty pounds during the initial month. Nevertheless, it is imperative to bear in mind that the consumption of creatine results in enhanced water retention within the human body. The increase in size that occurs from the consumption of creatine is partially a result of water retention, though the remaining portion consists solely of lean muscle mass. You will observe a significant increase in strength and a more pronounced muscular appearance.

Despite the endogenous production of creatine in the human body, its quantity is insufficient to yield any notable impact on your physical training. Creatine is also present in sources such as fresh meat, fish, cranberries, and other similar food items. Creatine exhibits a high degree of sensitivity towards elevated temperatures. Throughout the process of culinary preparation, it is highly probable that the integrity of creatine's structure will be compromised owing to the application of heat. This is why the usage of creatine supplementation holds significance in providing an amplified level of vigor and stamina to facilitate enhanced performance during physical exercise.

## Chapter One: Optimal Nutrition for Enhancing Muscular Development!

Numerous individuals engaged in bodybuilding often profess adherence to a unique (occasionally clandestine) dietary regimen, enabling them to sustain their impeccable physique. Notwithstanding the intricacy and challenge entailed by these dietary plans, it is noteworthy that they commonly encompass identical categories of food groups, which should not be limited to solely protein-based sources. Presented herewith is an inventory detailing the 15 most commendable food items that are highly recommended for inclusion in one's diet, with the objective of attaining the revered Adonis physique.

Let's start!

Wheat germ. Allow us to commence by introducing a food product that harbors merely negligible quantities of protein, yet possesses an inherent indispensability in the diets of individuals who engage in bodybuilding. Wheat germ contains a rich assortment of essential nutrients, including BCAAs (branched-chain amino acids), glutamine, arginine, potassium, selenium, zinc, iron, fiber, and energizing B-vitamins. This renders wheat germ as an ideal and optimal source of carbohydrates, offering a steady supply of energy that is gradually metabolized. They also encompass an abundance of foundational elements of protein, making them an ideal choice for consumption just prior to your exercise session.

Ezekial 4:9 bread. This particular food product is highly obscure in domains beyond the sphere of bodybuilding, health, and fitness. Nonetheless, it has the potential to yield remarkable results regardless of the dietary regimen followed. Ezekial 4:9 bread, which is crafted from sprouted organic whole grains as opposed to just regular whole grain, can be found in the majority of health stores. Due to its composition comprising both legumes and grains, the bread essentially qualifies as a comprehensive source of protein. In other words, it encompasses all nine indispensable amino acids that the human body is incapable of synthesizing independently, particularly those significant for the development of lean muscle mass.

Greek yogurt. Greek yogurt distinguishes itself from regular yogurt by presenting an exceptional nutritional profile, boasting a remarkable 20 grams of protein in a single cup while remaining derived from the same fundamental ingredient, milk. Incorporate that with its low carbohydrate content (approximately 9 grams per cup), rendering it a highly nutritious food for muscle development that also possesses exceptional flavor! This stands in contrast to the regular yogurt, which contains 16 grams of both protein and carbohydrates per cup. Greek yogurt is also an excellent provider of casein protein, notably contributing to enhanced muscle preservation and heightened reduction of body fat.

Apples. Is it not true that the consumption of one apple per day has the adage of preventing the need for medical intervention? However, it is not widely known that apples also contribute to physical fitness and body composition. The presence of polyphenols in apples imparts benefits such as enhanced muscular strength and reduced muscle fatigue. In essence, it can assist in augmenting your training intensity and duration. Additionally, there have been studies that suggest the potential fat-burning properties of polyphenols. Due to this fact, apples serve as excellent sources of carbohydrates prior to a workout.

Spinach. Remember Popeye? Indeed, it appears that his extensive inclination towards consuming spinach possesses a scientific rationale. This vegetable serves as a superior provider of amino acids and glutamine, effectively facilitating the muscular development towards a more toned physique. Similar to the mariner, it is also capable of enhancing one's muscular strength and endurance.

Wonka's Pixy Stix brand confectionery. Indeed, it is the confectionery. Why? Due to the presence of dextrose, an immediately available source of carbohydrates that requires no digestion, Pixy Stix possess this characteristic. Dextrose is capable of direct absorption into the bloodstream, bypassing physiological barriers, and promptly delivering vital nutrients to the muscles, which facilitates the optimal and expedient recovery process.

Moreover, it offers the additional appeal of a diverse range of flavors.

Quinoa. This particular grain has become notably recognized as a nourishing dietary option in contemporary times, and for valid reasons. Besides its ability to be digested gradually and its significant protein content, quinoa has also been associated with an elevation in insulin-like growth factor-1 (IGF-1). IGF-1 has been associated with strength and lean muscle gains.

Organic milk. Indeed, all organic items are significantly superior. Organic milk exhibits an increase of up to 70% in omega-3 fatty acid content when compared to its conventionally-produced counterpart. Similar to conventional milk, it comprises both whey and casein, alongside a notable abundance of glutamine.

Eggs. Similar to the method used by Rocky, increasing your consumption of eggs could be highly beneficial in your pursuit of bodybuilding efforts. This particular food item is widely recognized as the "optimal source of protein" for facilitating muscle development. However, it is often overlooked that this attribute is not solely attributable to protein content. The protein composition of an egg is enhanced by the yolk, which is also the source of cholesterol. Are you considering the status of your cholesterol levels? Based on scholarly investigations, studies have demonstrated that eggs possess the potential to effectively reduce the presence of LDL (low-density lipoproteins, colloquially referred to as "bad cholesterol"). This reduction is particularly significant as it is linked with the development of atherosclerosis.

Cottage cheese. Although excessive consumption of traditional processed cheese can have negative impacts on one's overall health, incorporating cottage cheese into one's diet can contribute to the development and strengthening of muscles. It contains a substantial amount of casein protein, which plays a crucial role in preserving muscle tissue by preventing their utilization as an energy source during the body's nocturnal reparative processes. Consequently, cottage cheese serves as an optimal pre-bedtime snack choice for individuals engaged in bodybuilding activities.

Cantaloupe. This particular melon belongs to a limited selection of fruits renowned for their capacity to function as expeditious sources of carbohydrates during digestion. This is due to its comparatively low fructose content. This renders the cantaloupe an excellent option to consume as a morning staple, following a prolonged period of abstinence throughout the night. This fruit, in addition, belongs to the limited selection of fruits that remains highly suitable for consumption even in the aftermath of physical exertion.

Oranges. The consumption of oranges prior to exercise has been purported to enhance muscle development, augmenting both its potency and resilience.

Brown Rice. While all types of whole grains are beneficial, brown rice distinguishes itself by virtue of its slow-digesting properties, which facilitate the provision of sustained energy during your workout and even thereafter. Furthermore, the consumption of brown rice can also contribute to the elevation of growth hormones (GH) levels, thereby promoting the reduction of body fat, enhancement of muscular strength, and development of lean muscle mass.

Beets. For individuals with a preference for root crops, it is noteworthy to ascertain that not all of these possess starch content. Beets serve as a valuable reservoir of betaine, a naturally occurring compound recognized alternatively as trimethylglycine. This dietary component not only facilitates the augmentation of muscular strength and power, but also promotes the improvement of liver and joint restoration. In addition, beets possess the ability to augment the energy levels of individuals engaging in bodybuilding activities and facilitate their recovery process, particularly following intense and arduous exercise sessions.

Beef. An alternative phrase in a formal tone: "Another culinary item held in high regard by the bodybuilding community, individuals seeking to develop their musculature are advised to consume not simply any variety of beef, but specifically that derived from grass-fed bovine sources." Beef constitutes a rich amalgamation of nutrients that are beneficial for muscle health, encompassing protein, cholesterol (similar to that found in eggs), B vitamins, zinc, and iron. Furthermore, beef sourced from grass-fed cattle possesses an elevated concentration of CLA (conjugated linoleic acid), aiding in the process of reducing body fat and promoting the development of lean muscle mass.

# Basics of Bodybuilding Nutrition

Proper nutrition plays a pivotal role in the attainment of success in bodybuilding. If one is truly committed and determined to attain their desired physique, it is imperative to adhere to a well-balanced and nutritious dietary regimen. Below are some of the nutrition tips that you can follow as you inch your way to bodybuilding success.

Protein Intake

A crucial component of a bodybuilding dietary regimen is the adequate consumption of a substantial amount of protein. The suggested amount is one gram of protein per pound of bodyweight per day, with the option to increase to a maximum of two grams per pound for individuals with difficulties in gaining muscle mass. Protein needs differ between individuals, however, by ensuring a minimum intake, one can effectively promote the growth of muscle mass.

All categories of protein are beneficial for bodybuilders aiming to increase their muscle mass. Nevertheless, lean meat, such as chicken, beef, and turkey, constitutes the most preferable choice. It is advisable to incorporate animal protein in each meal, striving to include lean varieties of red meat whenever feasible.

Fish serves as a highly commendable protein-rich food source that ought to be incorporated into the regular diet of bodybuilders. Certain varieties of fish contain significant amounts of beneficial fats, whereas others possess minimal levels of fat content. Nevertheless, fish with high fatty acid content is good for a bodybuilder.

Dairy and eggs are equally advantageous sources of protein. Additionally, they are more cost-effective. Ensure that when consuming eggs, one opts exclusively for the egg whites should they desire a protein source that is low in calories. The egg yolks serve as a beneficial source of healthy fats.

Carbohydrate Intake

When engaging in vigorous training, the consumption of carbohydrates assumes critical significance, as they serve as a primary source of fuel for the body, enabling proteins and fats to be directed towards accomplishing distinct objectives. Emphasize the inclusion of slow-digesting carbohydrates and whole-grain products in your diet, as they have the potential to yield sustained energy and are less likely to be stored as adipose tissue.

In order to increase your muscle mass effectively, it is essential to consume a daily intake of 2-3 grams of carbohydrates per pound of body weight. During the cutting phase, it is advised to decrease your carbohydrate consumption to 1 gram per pound of body weight.

Reduce consumption of simple carbohydrates as they are swiftly absorbed by the body. An excessive amount of simple carbohydrates can be readily converted into adipose tissue and stored in the body.

Saturated Fat vs. Trans Fats

Excessive consumption of these two types of fats can heighten the likelihood of developing heart disease and various other health complications. They can impede your progress in bodybuilding as well. Saturated and trans fats are commonly present in processed food items and baked products.

Nevertheless, there exist a category of beneficial fats known as unsaturated fats, which prove to be highly advantageous for individuals engaged in bodybuilding. There exists a prevalent misconception that a diet tailored for bodybuilding necessitates a reduction in fat intake. This statement is inaccurate - the dietary regimen should consist of reduced levels of trans and saturated fats.

Omega-3 fatty acids present in fish offer notable health benefits by creating an optimal condition for muscle development and sustaining a lean physique.

Calorie Count

Take note of the cumulative caloric consumption within a 24-hour period. It is imperative to maintain a diet that offers proper balance. In order to effectively increase your muscle mass, it is necessary to ensure that your dietary intake is a minimum of 20 calories per pound of body weight. If your objective is to maintain a lean physique, it is recommended to limit your caloric intake to 15 pounds per pound of bodyweight.

Drink Plenty of Water

Water is life. Adequate hydration is crucial for maintaining optimal health and can contribute positively to the process of muscular development. Ensure proper hydration by consuming a minimum of one gallon of water per day. Water is instrumental in facilitating protein synthesis and promoting efficient digestion. By continuously maintaining proper hydration, one can ensure a constant and uninterrupted flow of nutrients through the bloodstream, facilitating their delivery to the muscles.

Water plays a crucial role in maintaining muscle fullness and promoting the preservation of lean body mass, rendering it of particular significance to all individuals, particularly those engaged in bodybuilding.

Fiber

The majority of the foods endorsed in bodybuilding are characterized by a low fiber content. Nevertheless, bodybuilders require a substantial quantity of dietary fiber in order to attain optimal muscle growth. Consume a sufficient amount of dietary fiber, particularly if you are following a high-calorie eating regimen.

Grains and Starches

In general, it is recommended to incorporate grains into your bodybuilding regimen; however, it is crucial to be mindful of the impact they may have on your physique. Certain bodybuilders remain relatively unaffected by their daily consumption of grains and starches, whereas others must diligently regulate their dietary intake. Nevertheless, it is imperative for every bodybuilder to opt for whole-grain alternatives rather than processed options.

Fruits and Vegetables

Fruits and vegetables are highly valuable as dietary sources of fiber. They possess a rich array of nutrients that can support the development of muscle mass while promoting a lean physique. In order to fulfill the body's requirements, it is imperative for bodybuilders to strive for a daily consumption of five to six servings of vegetables.

Fruits, conversely, provide antioxidants and serve as commendable sources of dietary fiber and carbohydrates. The majority of fruits consist of slow-digesting carbohydrates, thereby providing an increased level of energy.

Bodybuilding Supplements

Nutritional supplements are integral to one's bodybuilding regimen, acting in synergy with the entirety of their dietary plan. These supplements can assist you in achieving your objective, however, it is important to bear in mind that they do not possess the power to instantaneously fulfill your desires. It is imperative that one possesses the knowledge and proficiency to utilize supplements judiciously and have a clear understanding of the anticipated outcomes they can offer. If you diligently adhere to a rigorous exercise routine and follow the prescribed supplement regimen, you will unquestionably achieve the desired outcomes.

Protein Supplements

Consume protein supplements a minimum of once per day on days of rest, and subsequently increase intake to twice daily on days dedicated to physical exercise. By opting for a reputable protein supplement brand, it is possible to fulfill your daily protein intake requirements. This dietary supplement has the potential to accelerate the process of muscle growth, and discernible advancements can be observed within a span of merely four months. In order to optimize the full potential of a protein supplement, it is imperative that your dietary intake is characterized by a high protein content while maintaining a low caloric value.

## Creatine

Creatine confers numerous advantages, such as expediting recuperation following rigorous exercise, reducing muscular soreness, and augmenting both muscle mass and strength. Consume an amount of creatine ranging from 3 to 5 grams prior to commencing your exercise routine and again afterwards.

## Arginine

Arginine is commonly incorporated into the supplementation regime of bodybuilders. This imperative amino acid possesses the capacity to enhance the secretion of growth hormones. This has the potential to accelerate the process of wound healing and provide significant post-workout benefits for the body. Additionally, arginine has the capacity to enhance muscle growth and strength by promoting increased blood flow.

Glucosamine and Chondroitin

Glucosamine plays a crucial role in supporting the health of cartilage, while chondroitin serves as the principal constituent of connective tissues and cartilages. This combination is frequently encountered in a singular supplement and is utilized by individuals engaged in bodybuilding for both the treatment and prevention of joint injuries.

Vitamin C

This potent antioxidant possesses the capacity to facilitate the process of hormone synthesis. It possesses the capability to enhance the immune system's functionality and mitigate potential damage.

## Vitamin E

This antioxidant possesses the ability to prolong the lifespan of erythrocytes and contributes to the preservation of bodily tissues.

## Glutamine

This is recognized for enhancing an individual's immune system and serves as a crucial amino acid for bodybuilders.

## Strategies and Techniques for Building Muscle through Diet

In order to assist you in achieving your bodybuilding objectives, it is imperative that you acquire proficiency in several efficacious approaches. If you have been engaged in the pursuit of bodybuilding for an extended period of time, it is possible that there are certain elements or misconceptions that have eluded your understanding. Presented herewith are a set of recommendations and strategies pertaining to the dietary regimen of a bodybuilder.

Big Breakfast

A substantial morning meal is imperative for individuals engaged in bodybuilding. Regardless of whether one is aiming to increase muscle mass or reduce body fat, it is imperative that the breakfast meal contains an ample amount of complex carbohydrates and protein. Consuming a substantial breakfast has the potential to initiate physiological processes, enabling the assimilation of vital nutrients and energy required for sustained vitality during the entirety of the day.

Eat Many Meals

It is imperative for bodybuilders to consume a minimum of 5 meals on rest days and a total of 7 meals on days when they engage in workouts. Consuming multiple meals conveys a consistent supply of vital nutrients to the body, facilitating the process of muscle development. The consistent provision of calories sustains your metabolic rate, thereby facilitating energy expenditure and preventing the accumulation of body fat.

Protein in Every Meal

In addition to consuming multiple meals throughout the day, it is important to ensure a sufficient intake of protein during each of these meals. Ensure that you are consuming a minimum of 20 grams of protein per meal. The consistent provision of protein will help to prevent the depletion of muscle tissues in your body.

## Pre-workout Meal

It is advisable to consume a light meal prior to engaging in physical exercise, as this can contribute to enhancing your energy levels and facilitate the recovery process following your workout.

## Post-Workout Meals

Post-exercise meals are comprised of two components. This particular time frame holds significant significance as it allows for the efficient replenishment of glycogen stores in the body by swiftly digesting carbohydrates following a workout. The initial step involves consumi

Following the completion of your training session, or approximately one hour later, consume a substantial protein-rich solid meal. It has the potential to facilitate the process of recuperation and promote the development of muscular tissues.

## Do Not Go Hungry

Even if your objective is to diminish body fat, it is advisable to refrain from experiencing hunger. It is advisable not to defer consumption until the onset of hunger, as this practice depletes muscle reserves by converting them into energy.

11. The utilization of hexagonal bars may provide a distinct benefit to your performance in deadlift exercises.

The dead lift is an essential component of weightlifting, despite experiencing some decline in popularity in recent times. In essence, the utilization of machines and other weightlifting aids essentially deprives one of the authentic toil inherent in weightlifting. In the context of a dead lift, one is either capable of lifting the weight or not. It is predicated upon innate physical power. Taking that into consideration, let us examine the benefits that a hexagonal bar might present to weightlifters who are interested in incorporating the deadlift into their routines. They\\\'re definitely worth considering.

To commence, the hexagonal bar, as implied by its name, is skillfully forged into a geometric shape known as a hexagon, featuring conveniently positioned hand grips adjacent to the inner collar of said bar. Due to the utilization of the hex bar, the lifting of weight is made feasible in a standing position, thereby eliminating the necessity of a bench or any auxiliary equipment. As a result of the hex bar's design, the barbell is positioned approximately parallel to your hips, alleviating the issue encountered with conventional weights where your legs often obstruct movement. Therefore, the weight is more centrally located within your body mass, resulting in a more uniform distribution throughout your legs and upper body. The primary benefit associated with the hexagonal bar resides in its ability to significantly reduce the burden and strain exerted on one's back. This attribute proves exceedingly advantageous, as injuries related to the spine can result in a prolonged cessation of weightlifting activities. Consequently, numerous professional weightlifters incline towards resorting to the hex bar during the execution of deadlifts, or at the very least, exclusively utilizing the straight-bar when not in a competitive period.

The design additionally ensures that the hexagonal bar is more accommodating for individuals with a previous medical history of chronic back pain, as compared to the straight-bar alternative. Consequently, this enables them to engage in deadlifting without apprehension of aggravating prior injuries. An understandable relief!

## 16. The Treadmill: A Pathway Towards Cardiovascular Wellness

The impending arrival of the new year coincides with the commitment you will make to engage in a jogging routine. However, running through the cold, snow-covered streets does not offer a pleasant encounter. Furthermore, it is exceedingly challenging and potentially hazardous to inhale the frigid atmosphere. One noteworthy approach to address this particular circumstance is to utilize a treadmill. For certain individuals, undoubtedly, this alternative may not be deemed an acceptable substitute to the customary notion of "fresh" air. Nevertheless, I venture to assert that the quality of air within urban environments is scarcely fresh. Therefore, both your cardiovascular system and pulmonary system will express gratitude for the decision to engage in this particular form of physical activity. To promote cardiovascular well-being, adhere to a handful of uncomplicated guidelines.

Incorporate running with resistance training.

Initially, it is imperative to commence with a brief warm-up session of approximately five minutes, conducted at a comfortable pace. Afterward, you may opt to enthusiastically discontinue the use of the treadmill and instead engage in a modest augmentation of intensity through a series of power exercises such as push-ups, sit-ups, tilts, and abdominal crunches. Following a session of weight training, it is advisable to take a brief respite of a few minutes before resuming activity on the treadmill. Please endeavor to complete four sets of both running and strength training exercises. However, it is important to bear in mind that excessive training is unnecessary. Commencing the exercise routine, individuals are instructed to perform a prescribed quantity of sets with repetitions, and, if required, adjust the quantity accordingly.

Incorporate variety in your cardio exercises by alternating the use of the treadmill with other activities.

Endeavor to incorporate treadmill workouts alongside other training modalities in order to facilitate cardiovascular development and fortification. In lieu of utilizing the treadmill, alternative options such as stationary bikes or elliptical trainers may be employed, as they proffer a well-rounded distribution of exertion across the chest, leg muscles, and cardiovascular system, naturally. If you engage in a 40-minute cardiovascular exercise routine, allocate 10 minutes to running on the treadmill and an additional 10 minutes to utilizing the alternative simulator. Continue your diligent efforts until you achieve the designated timeframe. If one engages in home-based physical activity and possesses only a treadmill as their sole sports equipment, it may be deemed appropriate to employ a standard step ladder as a viable alternative for additional cardiovascular exercise. During the intermissions between treadmill workout sessions, you may engage in a 5-minute self-paced activity of ascending and descending the stairs.

Utilize the enjoyment of music during your exercise routine.

Occasionally, the act of running on a treadmill can be dull as the stationary surroundings offer no variation, and the audio accompaniment is restricted solely to the synchronized hum of the machine, rhythmic footsteps, and breathing. In this particular situation, the most optimal course of action would be to listen to music of your preference. There are individuals who hold the opinion that engaging in music while running may compromise safety, as one needs to remain fully aware of their surroundings. However, this concern may not be applicable to individuals who engage in exercising within the confines of their homes. On the contrary, music has the potential to uplift one's mood, thereby contributing to the optimization of an effective weight loss routine. Generate your personalized playlist, which will serve as a source of motivation and enable you to monitor the duration of your exercise regimen as it progressively increases during regular training sessions.

Implementing rest periods following physical exertion

Maintain a consistent pace of running, without hesitating to engage in exploratory variations such as alternating between calm and accelerated running. This practice will enhance muscular endurance, subsequently fortifying the cardiovascular system. Following a brief five-minute warm-up, endeavor to engage in the three sets lasting four minutes each. Subsequently, take a moment to recuperate and permit your muscles to gradually return to their normal state.

Maintain a positive demeanor.

The paramount aspect of this physical activity is that it ought to be pleasurable and amenable for you to engage in exercise. There is no obligation to exert oneself while in a negative emotional state; in doing so, one can effortlessly achieve optimal outcomes.

## Skeletal Muscles

The muscular structures observed and palpated within the human body are referred to as skeletal muscles. These muscles are the ones that you will engage when seeking to enhance muscle mass. The integration of robust tendons with skeletal muscles serves to consolidate the physique, bestowing formidable strength and vigor to the entire body structure.

There exists a vast array of skeletal muscles within the human body; however, the principal and most well-recognized ones include:

Deltoid muscles can be located in the shoulder region. They facilitate the coordinated movement of your shoulders – encompassing actions such as swinging a golf club, propelling your arms during swimming, executing shoulder shrugs while dancing, as well as aiding in the removal of your jacket.

The rectus abdominus, colloquially referred to as the abdominal muscles, is situated beneath the ribcage. The attainment of a well-defined set of abdominal muscles, commonly referred to as "6-pack abs," is a highly desirable goal for individuals seeking physical fitness.

Pectoralis muscles are situated in the lateral region of the upper chest, also commonly referred to as pectorals or pecs. During adolescence, the pectoral muscles in males naturally experience an increase in size.

Gluteus maximus – The gluteus maximus muscles are located in the anatomical region known as the buttocks. If you desire to enhance the appearance of your buttocks to achieve a firm and aesthetically pleasing contour, engaging in exercises that target the gluteus maximus muscle can be efficacious.

Quadriceps – Have you ever observed the muscular development in the anterior region of the thighs of a runner or rugby player? These particular muscles are referred to as the quadriceps or quadricep muscles.

The biceps muscle is widely recognized as one of the most prominent types of skeletal muscles. Located in the upper extremities, this particular muscle exhibits a noticeable protrusion of the skin when the elbow is bent and contracted.

Skeletal Muscle Enlargement

Indeed, the growth of skeletal muscle parallels your own development. However, as individuals mature and experience a surge in testosterone levels, their skeletal muscles undergo an increase in size with relative ease, albeit not always externally evident.

The muscular tissue comprises a vast number of individual muscle cells or fibers. Slow twitch and fast twitch fibers serve as the respective classifications for these muscular strands. Slow twitch or Type I fibers possess a notable resistance to fatigue and possess the capability to metabolize oxygen into energy, allowing for prolonged engagement in aerobic exercises. Fast twitch or Type II fibers enable rapid movement, albeit with a propensity for quick fatigue.

There is variation in the proportion of slow twitch and fast twitch muscle fibers in your body compared to others. Hence, you may possess inherent aptitude for marathons over sprints, or exhibit superior proficiency in executing High

Interval Intensity (HIIT) sets rather than prolonged workout sessions.

In order to enhance the visibility and size of your muscles, it is necessary to increase the dimensions of these muscle fibers. The process of muscle fiber enlargement is referred to as hypertrophy.

Myofibril Hypertrophy concerns the augmentation of muscle fibers, with an emphasis on fortifying the contractile component of the muscle. It promotes enhanced muscular fiber densification and strengthening.

Sarcoplasmic hypertrophy accounts for approximately 30% of our muscle bulk, attributable to the presence of sarcoplasmic fluid within the muscular structure. Sarcoplasmic hypertrophy is centered around augmenting the volume of sarcoplasmic fluid, thereby facilitating significant enlargement of the muscular structure.

Temporary Hypertrophy – Referred to as a transient enlargement in muscle size, temporary hypertrophy manifests immediately subsequent to an intense resistance training session.

Given your objective to develop significant muscle mass, it is advisable to prioritize sarcoplasmic hypertrophy.

What is the impact on muscular tissues?" or "What is the physiological response of muscles?

During weightlifting, the musculature undergoes an automatic adaptation process, leading to an enlargement of the muscles in order to counteract and mitigate stress and strain. With the execution of each repetition of substantial resistance, the skeletal muscle fibers undergo micro-tears.

However, once that minuscule tear has repaired itself, the muscle will exhibit enhanced flexibility and strength, particularly through consistent repetition. This elucidates the ease with which you are able to handle the 50-pound dumbbell that previously posed significant challenge to you just a few months ago.

As one progressively augments repetitions and weight range, commensurate enlargement of muscles shall occur.

Why Lift Weights?

It is not obligatory for males to possess well-developed musculature – prominently defined biceps, robust lower limbs, and a taut abdominal region. However, it should be noted that possessing a well-defined, muscular physique can attract the interest of both women and men. If you happen to be of a youthful age, pursuing modeling or acting can potentially enhance your chances of securing employment in these fields, should you have an inclination towards them.

Individuals who aspire to attain significant muscular development possess varying motives for their pursuit. However, they all share a collective aim: to project an unequivocal sense of masculinity. If you happen to be an individual seeking to augment your muscle mass, it is imperative for you to ascertain whether your desired outcome leans towards achieving a physique akin to the impeccably chiseled and refined constitution exuded by Henry Cavill as Superman, the immense and well-defined presence personified by Dwayne "The Rock" Johnson, or the awe-inspiring power and physical prowess exhibited by the reigning World's Strongest Man. It may prove to be challenging and time-consuming, albeit feasible. For those who are inclined to maximize their muscularity, kindly direct your attention to the subsequent chapter.

Exercise Selection

All right then. At this point, it is expected that you have thoroughly assessed your exercise catalog and have developed a tentative understanding regarding the frequency and intensity of training desired for each muscle group. Now is the opportune moment to apply the exercises you have acquired with proficiency.

You can achieve this by populating the muscle group slots in your program framework with appropriate and targeted exercises. Thus, let us take the chest as an illustrative example.

Typically, a range of two to four exercises proves to be sufficient for a frequency of two to three weekly sessions targeting each muscle group. In contrast to prevailing conjecture, a plethora of diverse exercises is not an imperative element in optimizing hypertrophy. An excessive range of options can potentially have a detrimental effect, as it is crucial to maintain a certain level of specificity in your muscle-building training regimen in order to facilitate adaptations and ensure appropriate advancement. Additionally, should you include an excessive number of exercises in your program, it would result in wastage of significant time dedicated to warming up, relocating within the gym for training, and potentially waiting for machines or equipment to become available.

Furthermore, given that you may initially undertake exercises with a rather modest training volume, it is unnecessary to exceed the recommended limits. This holds especially true if your intention is to engage in muscle training three times per week, with an even lower volume per session. It would be rather inefficient to go through the process of warming up for the bench press, perform only one intense set, and then immediately transition to a different chest exercise that requires another warm-up. You would effectively allocate a greater amount of time to warming up than to actual training.

Regarding the exercise selection, commence by selecting a single high-impact primary exercise for each significant muscle group:

Upper body strength exercise, specifically the barbell overhead press.

Pectoral exercise (specifically, barbell bench press)

Assisted pull-ups, also known as back exercises...

Quads (i.e., squats)

Gluteus muscles and hamstrings (specifically, the Romanian deadlift).

Alternatively, it is imperative to incorporate all of the subsequent movements patterns.

Horizontal pressing exercise for the pectoral muscles.

Shoulder exercises for upward movement

Horizontal pulling exercise for the (upper) back

Vertical traction for (mid) dorsal area.

Hinge for hams/glutes

Squat for quads

Additionally, it would be desirable to include the following:

Shoulder lateral abduction for the development of the deltoid muscle on the side of the body

Triceps elbow extension

Elbow flexion to engage the biceps muscles.

Nevertheless, when targeting these smaller muscle groups, it may be advisable to consider isolation exercises as they can effectively target certain muscles that are difficult to fully engage with compound movements. As an illustration, one could potentially engage in chin-ups as a means to target their biceps; however, it is likely that the exertion would primarily be felt in the forearms or back muscles, rather than the desired bicep muscles. This is unfavorable information for individuals seeking to achieve optimal biceps growth. An exercise such as performing a weighted EZ-bar curl would likely yield more satisfactory results.

This is essential for any exercise you select with the goal of achieving hypertrophy. If the target muscle is not acting as the constraining element in your sets, you run the risk of their expenditure being futile. Approaching the point of failure (which will be addressed shortly) is another essential factor in the development of muscle.

Nonetheless, in the event that the exercise you have selected incites you to halt your sets for any purpose other than the targeted muscle's incapacity to sustain further effort, what rationale justifies your inclusion of said exercise in your routine? When selecting your exercises, it is imperative that you consistently inquire: "

What specific muscle should be considered as the determining factor of its limitations?

After selecting your main workout, it is likely to occupy a significant portion of your exercise routine dedicated to the respective muscle group, as excessive volume or extensive variations per workout are unnecessary at this stage, especially for individuals who are beginners.

However, it is important to note that a lack of need for excessive variation should not justify the adoption of an excessively narrow training regimen. As an illustration, engaging in bench presses consistently on Mondays, Wednesdays, and Fridays with the same repetition range is likely to result in missed opportunities for progress and rapidly diminishing effectiveness in chest training.

Therefore, to fill the remaining slot(s), it is recommended to select an additional primary or secondary compound exercise that employs distinct equipment (such as dumbbells instead of a barbell), a varying repetition range, and ideally targets the desired muscle group from a different perspective or with an altered resistance curve (for example, incline pressing instead of flat pressing for a different angle, or spider curls rather than standing EZ-bar curls for a distinct resistance curve). By doing so, you can achieve an ideal equilibrium, ensuring that your training remains engaging and diverse, while still maintaining its focus and targeted nature.

Revisiting our aforementioned analogy regarding the chest, this may entail performing a rigorous bench press routine on the initial day devoted to chest exercises, followed by a moderately intense session on the subsequent day involving dumbbell incline presses and, if desired, supplementary cable flys.

Regarding isolation exercises for the primary muscle groups, it would be advisable to incorporate one into your routine if you have sufficient capacity or if a particular muscle group necessitates it for optimal development. For the latter, the shoulders serve as a prime specimen, as the maximization of side deltoid development cannot be achieved solely through the execution of overhead pressing variations.

However, it is advisable to adhere to the two out of three or three out of four rule when incorporating isolation exercises for the primary muscle groups. Consequently, when selecting three exercises for your major muscle groups, it is advisable to choose two foundational or impactful exercises and one isolation exercise. Should you choose the number four, please select a combination of three primary or secondary exercises, as well as one isolation exercise.

However, it should be noted that this is merely a suggestion. Occasionally, it may not be necessary to engage in isolation exercises and instead dedicate one's attention solely to compound movements, as is the case with my current chest training regimen. It ultimately boils down to individual preferences and the amount of time one can allocate.

An additional rule to adhere to is to maintain your selection of exercises within the designated repetition ranges for a minimum of one mesocycle, and ideally for two or even a complete block of training. Engaging in frequent and varied exercise rotation without assessing your progression can be detrimental to hypertrophy outcomes, which is highly undesirable. Allow me to provide you with an illustration:

In the first week, the recommended regimen involves performing three sets of barbell bench presses at a weight of

135 lbs, completing 10 repetitions in the first set, 8 repetitions in the second set, and 7 repetitions in the third set.

In the second week, you will perform three sets of dumbbell incline presses instead, utilizing the 50-pound dumbbells for repetitions of 12, 10, and 8.

Inquiry: Did your chest performance demonstrate improvement, deterioration, or consistency in Week 2 as compared to Week 1?

Response: It is impossible to determine.

I would prefer not to jump too far ahead as I intend to delve into this topic extensively in the subsequent part dedicated to its progression. It is essential to recognize the significance of progressive overload in order to effectively promote muscle growth. The state of being unaware of one's progress is comparable to attempting to navigate from point A to point B while blinded. Certainly, you have the potential to reach that point with time and effort. However, it is also possible that you could become disoriented or encounter an obstacle such as a tree.

# Weight Training Principles You've Overlooked That's Stopping You From Building Crazy Muscle And Strength

## Progressive Overload

This is a principle that I have recently incorporated into my training regimen, and the results I have witnessed in the past year have surpassed those achieved over the preceding 5 years. I am notifying you in advance to prevent you from committing the same error as I did.

Progressive overload refers to the sustained elevation of resistance imposed on an individual's physique. As you progress in your training over time, it is clearly desirable to augment the resistance applied to your body, which may not exclusively involve the addition of weight. Progressive overload guarantees a perpetual increase in strength.

Failure to augment the resistance imposed on your physique will inevitably impede your capacity for strength development and muscle hypertrophy. By incorporating the principle of progressive overload, you can guarantee effective muscle development, substantial size gains, and enhanced physical strength. The augmentation in resistance can arise from various factors, including additional repetitions, greater weight load, increased number of sets, reduced rest intervals, and manipulation of tempo durations - all of which will be comprehensively discussed within the contents of this book.

Reps

It is expected that you possess a fundamental understanding of training principles. In the event that you do not possess this understanding, I will proceed to provide a succinct overview for your benefit. A single repetition denotes a solitary instance of executing the exercise. As an illustration, a single repetition is equivalent to performing one push-up. One repetition is completed with each singular pull-up. Capiche? If your goal is to enhance your strength, it is advised to engage in weightlifting within the repetition range of 1 to 5, using substantial amounts of weight. One may choose to augment the weight in order to offset the reduction in repetitions, thereby yielding substantial enhancements in strength.

For individuals seeking to maximize muscle growth, a rep range of 6-12 repetitions is highly recommended. You will experience substantial muscular stimulation, elevated heart rate, and efficient breakdown of muscle fibers for subsequent rebuilding with adequate nutrition and rest. However, it should be noted that one can indeed develop strength within the 6-12 repetition range, and similarly, muscle growth can be achieved within the 1-5 repetition range. Nevertheless, the most optimal outcomes in terms of strength training are typically attained using the 1-5 rep range, while the 6-12 rep range tends to yield more favorable results for muscle building.

Sets

Quick breakdown numero two-no. Suppose you aspire to execute 12 repetitions of the bench press exercise, repeating the process thrice while incorporating intermittent rest periods. Consequently, you will be performing the bench press exercise for 3 sets, with 12 repetitions in each set.

The ultimate determination of how many sets to include in your training regimen rests with you. Initially, when I commenced weightlifting, my entire exercise regimen consisted of a mere 15 sets. Currently, I engage in a range of 25-30 sets per workout. That is simply due to the fact that I have developed the necessary endurance to perform that number of sets, and moreover, I derive genuine pleasure from engaging in training activities. For individuals who are inexperienced in weightlifting, I suggest performing approximately 15-20 sets. For those at an intermediate proficiency level, it is advisable to aim for 20-25 sets. As for advanced weightlifters, it is recommended to engage in 25 sets or more.

Stretch and Contraction

Engaging in the bench press without attaining the requisite extent of pectoral muscle elongation at the lower point of the exercise and subsequent flexion at the upper point inevitably renders any perceived chest-targeting ineffective. I must acknowledge that my contemplation on this matter commenced merely at the onset of the year. Presently, I earnestly strive to diligently attain the desired extension and flexibility in the movement. Consider this: One might believe they are executing the bicep curls correctly, assuming that merely performing the motion is sufficient to achieve muscular stimulation. However, in reality, there is a possibility that one may not be effectively engaging the bicep and fully contracting it at the pinnacle of the movement.

## Resting Between Sets

Undeniably, this is a matter that I have only recently begun to monitor and have never meticulously quantified in previous years. I had not anticipated the significant influence that this would have on the exercise routine. Reducing the intervals of rest between sets not only results in a reduced duration of the workout, but also intensifies the strain on your body, thereby facilitating its fortification.

In the context of muscle development, it is advisable to observe a resting period of 45-90 seconds between sets in order to maximize results. This will help maintain an elevated heart rate and ensure consistent muscular contraction. If the objective is to enhance muscular strength, it would be advantageous to allocate a suitable amount of time until your body perceives a sense of readiness to proceed with the subsequent set. Certain individuals recommend taking a rest period of 2-5 minutes for enhancing physical strength. However, I would suggest listening to your body and choosing a rest duration that aligns with your specific needs and preferences.

Controlling Your Breathing

The impact of respiration on physical training is truly remarkable. I'm certain you have encountered some instances in videos where individuals lose consciousness due to a cessation of breathing during strenuous physical activity.

I will quickly provide a breakdown of the topic. It is advisable to regulate your respiration to optimize the effectiveness of the exercises you are engaging in.

Regrettably, I am unable to provide direct assistance regarding individualized breathing techniques. However, it is commonly advised to inhale during the eccentric phase of the movement, while exhaling during the concentric phase of the movement. An illustration of this is evident in the execution of a squat movement, wherein inhalation is advised during the descent into a deep squat position, followed by exhalation when ascending to an upright stance. One can enhance their energy levels by performing a few deep breaths upon reaching the summit, followed by a subsequent descent. Above all, it is imperative to breathe at the appropriate moments.

Relieving Muscle Tension

Following extensive resistance training, the musculature undergoes noticeable tensing and the formation of knots, particularly in the upper back and neck regions. It is essential to alleviate all tension to optimize blood circulation within the muscles, and quite frankly, it provides a highly gratifying sensation.

There are alternative approaches to alleviate muscle tension, one of which involves engaging a professional massage therapist. However, it is worth noting that the services of a qualified practitioner can be quite expensive and may not align with one's budget or time constraints. The second alternative is to undertake the task independently. One can engage in self-application of the tennis ball massage technique and employ a foam roller as well. Both methods are cost-effective means by which you can alleviate muscular tightness in order to enhance your exercise regimen.

## Super Sets

Super sets constitute a technique used to stimulate muscle growth and enhance vascularity, involving the completion of Exercise A followed promptly by Exercise B within a single set. As an illustration, if you are engaged in a Chest/Back exercise regimen, you may opt to perform one set of incline bench press immediately succeeded by a set of pullups. This expedites the duration of the exercise regimen, enhances the efficacy of your workout, and also provides a notable muscular exertion within your upper physique. It is fairly straightforward; simply choose two exercises that you would like to perform simultaneously. Execute the superset followed by a subsequent cessation subsequent to the second exercise. In the context of a chest and shoulders workout, one may consider performing the flat barbell bench press, subsequently followed by a set of dips. If one is engaged in an upper body strength training session, one could potentially perform a series of barbell curls and subsequently execute a set of triceps pushups. The possibilities for exercise combinations are abundant and varied.

Drop sets

An esteemed choice of mine. A drop set involves performing an exercise until reaching muscular failure, subsequently reducing the weight load, and proceeding to execute a few additional repetitions until once again reaching the point of failure. Take, for instance, the scenario in which you are executing a bench press exercise with a weight of 220 pounds on the flat barbell. Should you desire to achieve an intensified muscle pump, a potential approach would be to decrease the weight to approximately 185 pounds and proceed to perform an additional set until reaching the point of muscular failure. By adopting this method, you can effectively stimulate and enhance muscle development in the chest and triceps, thereby facilitating further gains. Attention: Drop sets can be exceptionally challenging, yet they deliver a satisfying sensation and lead to substantial muscular growth.

Pyramid Sets

The pyramid entails commencing with a relatively low weight for x repetitions, followed by subsequent sets that progressively raise the weight and complete y repetitions, with this sequence being iterated. As an illustration, it is possible to perform one set of 10 repetitions using an 80-pound barbell for rows, followed by the subsequent set of 8 repetitions utilizing a 100-pound barbell, and then progressing to a set of 6 reps with a 120-pound barbell. This pattern can be continued accordingly. By adopting this approach, you will effectively diversify your workout regimen and stimulate your body to achieve substantial increases in both strength and muscle mass.

## Supplements

While the consumption of nourishing foods is beneficial, there exist supplementary options that can facilitate your weight training progression. Ranging from the fundamental multivitamin to more sophisticated supplements, we present a concise handbook outlining the ones you should contemplate incorporating into your regimen if your aim is to pursue a career as a female bodybuilder. Please be advised that the aforementioned points are simply offered as suggestions. It is not necessary to acquire all the supplements or equipment we recommend.

## Multivitamin

If you are not currently incorporating a multivitamin into your daily routine, we strongly recommend considering it. These contain essential nutrients that are potentially lacking in your dietary intake. These products are particularly beneficial for women with deficiencies in iron, vitamin B12, and folate. It is advisable to conduct thorough research prior to visiting the store, as the dosage of the multivitamin may differ depending on the specific brand.

Fish Oil

Several scientific investigations have yielded the finding that individuals can experience advantageous effects through the consumption of Omega-3 fatty acids derived from fish oil supplements. These fatty acids play a crucial role in the enhancement of cognitive development and the overall well-being of individuals. Based on certain studies, it has been determined that the consumption of fish oil exhibits the potential to mitigate the likelihood of certain types of cancers, while also effectively managing chronic inflammation. Given the multitude of advantages it encompasses, fish oil is generally deemed safe for the majority of individuals and can exclusively contribute to the enhancement of one's physical well-being.

Protein

As previously stated, if your intention is to cultivate additional lean mass, it is imperative that you supply adequate protein to support this process. If you are experiencing fatigue from the consumption of poultry, consider incorporating a protein shake into your dietary regimen. In addition to their convenient nature, the shakes possess a delightful taste and boast a protein content of up to 25 grams. Moreover, apart from this approach, there are alternative recipes available that enable the incorporation of protein into your daily meals through baking or blending.

## Probiotics

If you are not yet aware, there exists both beneficial and harmful bacteria. Fortunately, the presence of beneficial bacteria in our bodies is the underlying cause behind our ability to effectively metabolize food and assimilate essential nutrients. By consuming probiotics, you are promoting the acquisition of beneficial bacteria necessary for optimal bodily function. Search for food items such as kefir and yogurt that encompass Lactobacillus or Bifidobacterium. Supplemental forms of probiotics are available as well; nonetheless, it is imperative to ensure their origin from a reputable manufacturer. It is imperative to exercise caution and discretion in selecting substances to introduce into one's system, as failure to do so can potentially yield severe consequences.

## BCAAs

It is likely that you have encountered this term being used widely. BCAAs is an acronym that represents branched chain amino acids. In essence, the aforementioned protein blocks consist of leucine, isoleucine, and valine. They constitute the amino acids responsible for facilitating protein synthesis and enhancing post-workout recuperation.

What is the recommended frequency and duration per week for utilizing your gym exercise and fitness equipment?

Having acquired knowledge regarding the essential home accessories and bodybuilding equipment, as well as comprehending the optimal methods of utilizing them, the subsequent inquiry arises as to what duration should be allocated for such activities?

A crucial aspect of being knowledgeable about bodybuilding entails recognizing the frequency with which gadgets and accessories are consistently swapped and utilized by accomplished bodybuilders. It is essential to comprehend that his ability to consistently and strenuously exert himself, along with his relentless pursuit of additional resources, is not indicative of a frivolous disposition toward finances.

What is the recommended frequency of exercise for individuals engaged in bodybuilding?

How often have you engaged in gym memberships or committed to endeavors aimed at weight loss, only to abandon them a few weeks later due to a lack of understanding regarding the appropriate frequency of training?

If your response remains consistent, then you are in esteemed company. Understanding the appropriate duration for physical activity can be perplexing. This is especially true if the timeframe in which you are engaged does not align with your objectives.

Therefore, irrespective of whether your intention is to increase your frequency of treadmill sessions in order to lose a few pounds or to enhance the amount of weight you are lifting during a bulk phase, the following guidelines can assist you in achieving your goal more expeditiously and with more substantial advancements.

What is the recommended frequency of training when aiming to reduce body fat?

The frequency at which you engage in strength exercises and cardiovascular activities in order to achieve weight loss goals is contingent upon the speed at which you desire to attain results.

The overarching proposition is to aim for a gradual weight reduction of approximately 1 to 2 pounds per week. Taking all factors into account, a considerable number of individuals seek out programs specifically designed for expedited weight loss.

In the simplest of terms, the process of losing weight requires expending a greater amount of calories than you consume. Research has substantiated the efficacy of calorie counting as a viable approach to achieving weight loss goals. Nevertheless, in order to maintain weight reduction, it is imperative to engage in regular physical exercise.

The extent to which you can effectively lose weight depends on the level of physical activity you are willing to engage in and the degree to which you faithfully adhere to your dietary regimen. If you have a genuine concern for achieving outcomes that will manifest on a significant level and continue to progress consistently, it is imperative to devote your attention to exercising a minimum of four to five days per week." "Should you prioritize the attainment of consequential results that demonstrate notable growth over an extended period, it is essential to dedicate a minimum of four to five days each week to your workout routine." "If your objective is to obtain results that will have a significant impact and steadily advance over time, it is crucial to maintain a focus on engaging in workouts for a minimum of four to five days per week.

However, it is important to remember that you will progress towards this. To commence, it may be necessary to allocate several days per week and progressively increase the frequency to encompass a period of up to five days. Strategically structure your workout regimen to encompass a mixture of:

•Cardio

•Strength preparing

•Core work

•Stretching

For optimal results, an exercise regimen should consist of both cardiovascular and strength training exercises. When engaging in bodybuilding, the process of increasing your 'lean muscle mass' facilitates the enhancement of your metabolism, resulting in a heightened ability to burn calories even while at rest.

Engaging in cardiovascular exercise is not solely vital for maintaining optimal heart health. Engaging in cardiovascular exercises contributes to:

•burn calories

• enhance your demeanor • elevate your composure • improve your disposition • enhance your character • refine your behavior

•decrease stress

Presented herewith is the Cardiovascular exercise.

It is advisable for you to try either:

• Engage in 30 minutes of moderate-intensity cardiovascular exercise for a minimum of five days per week (amounting to a total of 150 minutes in a week)

•A minimum duration of 25 minutes per session, involving vigorous, high-impact physical activity, should be pursued three days per week, aggregating to a total of 75 minutes on a weekly basis.

In order to reduce body fat, it is advisable to incorporate two days of moderate-intensity exercise and two days of high-intensity interval training (HIIT) into your fitness routine.

Strength training

Direct your attention towards a select few days out of the comprehensive week-long preparation phase dedicated to fostering unity and collaboration.

Integrate comprehensive workout routines that prioritize compound movements. These movements engage various muscle groups simultaneously. Models include:

• Performing squats while executing a shoulder press • Engaging in a combination of squats and shoulder presses • Integrating squats and shoulder presses in one fluid movement

• Perform a deadlift while pivoting around the support column.

• Perform lunges while simultaneously executing a horizontal raise.

•Pushups and board with a one-arm column

Additional important elements to consider for your solidarity training program encompass:

- Squats

- Lunges

- Planks

- Pushups

- Straight-legged deadlifts

- Bench-presses

- Pushup plunges

- Overhead presses

- Pullups

- Dumbbell columns

- Planks

- Crunches using an exercise ball

In order to derive optimum advantages from your weight reduction exercises, it is imperative that you adhere to the following guidelines:

•Adjust the intensity of your exercises. Integrate both high-intensity interval training (HIIT) and exercises of moderate intensity.

•Execute a diverse range of cardiovascular exercises over the span of one week, including activities such as utilizing the treadmill, engaging in hiking expeditions, and partaking in swimming sessions.

• Employ circuit training as a means of effectively and consistently expending calories during your workout sessions. The circuit training regimen comprises a sequence of exercises performed continuously, without any intervals for rest between each exercise. At the culmination of the sequences of exercises, it is customary to engage in a predetermined period of rest (typically lasting between 30 to 60 seconds), after which you proceed to repeat the circuit on multiple occasions.

• It is recommended to allocate a minimum of 2 days per week for rest.

The subsequent inquiry that you are posing is, "

**Pick your carbs wisely.**

Carbohydrates are the foundational constituents of food, and comprehending their mechanisms will facilitate wise selection of nutrient sources to effectively support weight reduction and enhance the development of lean muscle.

The Conversion of Carbohydrates into Energy

Upon digestion of carbohydrates, enzymatic processes facilitate their conversion into sugars, subsequently leading to a rise in the blood glucose level. During this process, the pancreas secretes insulin, an anabolic hormone that facilitates the transportation of nutrients into muscle cells and aids in muscle recovery. The second role of insulin involves the disposal of excess glucose from the bloodstream by facilitating its transportation into the storage reserves of liver glycogen or muscle glycogen. Nevertheless, in the event that the glycogen reserves in the liver and muscles have reached their peak capacity, any excess glucose circulating in the bloodstream will be subsequently converted into adipose tissue.

During physical activity, the body utilizes its muscle glycogen stores, and the subsequent release of insulin triggered by the consumption of high-carbohydrate foods facilitates the transportation of excessive blood glucose, alongside other nutrients, into the muscle cells. This promotes enhanced muscle protein synthesis and facilitates efficient muscle recovery, ultimately resulting in the development of lean muscle mass.

As you are aware, that is your ultimate objective. You are engaging in these exercises with the ultimate goal of developing lean muscles. After establishing your goals, it becomes progressively more convenient for you to adhere to and strive towards them. Therefore, it is crucial to maximize the execution of correct actions in order to expedite the achievement of your objective. Exercise prudence when making decisions regarding the ingestion of carbohydrates. A more formal way to express the same idea would be: "Further elaboration on this matter can be found in the subsequent section."

The Significance of both Quantity and Quality
The extent to which your blood sugar rises due to carbohydrate intake is predominantly determined by the quantity consumed and the rate at which the carbohydrates are metabolized. The fiber content in carbohydrates, along with the levels of fat and protein, also constitutes a significant determinant.
To achieve weight loss and enhance muscle recovery through carbohydrate intake, it is advisable to opt for food sources that are not refined and possess a high fiber content. This will guarantee that the carbohydrate will undergo slower digestion, resulting in a more gradual elevation of blood sugar levels

and an insulin response that is more consistent. Processed carbohydrates and sugars, from which dietary fiber has been eliminated, are readily metabolized and cause a rapid increase in blood sugar levels, followed by a subsequent decline once insulin is released. Individuals who partake in the consumption of refined and processed carbohydrates such as white sugar, bread, and pasta often experience an intensified yearning for these foods due to the fluctuation in energy levels caused by the "spike and crash" pattern, consequently resulting in an increase in body weight. Thus, therein lies the crux of the entire matter. Numerous individuals attribute the habitual nature of their dietary choices to their staple foods.

Furthermore, unrefined carbohydrates not only contribute to a more even elevation of blood sugar levels and a steady insulin response, but they also offer a higher content of vitamins and minerals compared to refined carbohydrates, as the refining process often leads to the elimination of these crucial nutrients. Unprocessed carbohydrates encompass various whole grains, including brown rice, oatmeal, whole wheat, and bran; legumes, such as soybeans, peas, lentils, and peanuts; fruits, such as apples, strawberries, oranges, and grapes; and raw vegetables, such as broccoli, carrots, and spinach.

The Dietary Glycemic Index: A Comprehensive Investigation into the Impact of Food

The glycemic index, also known as GI, pertains to the classification of foods, specifically those that contain carbohydrates, into three distinct categories: low, medium, and high. Foods that elicit an instantaneous surge in blood sugar levels are classified as possessing a higher glycemic index, whereas foods that prompt a gradual elevation in blood sugar levels are characterized by a lower glycemic index. There exist numerous dietary regimens that incorporate the concept of the glycemic index (GI) as a means of identifying the fundamental nutritional categories of food to facilitate weight loss and long-term weight management. Therefore, it is of utmost importance for you to be mindful of your dietary choices when embarking on your lean muscle-building regimen.

The subsequent frequently consumed food items can be categorized as having a low glycemic index: a considerable variety of fruits and vegetables, a significant portion of dairy products, sweet potatoes, whole and unprocessed grains, legumes, and barley.

The high GI category includes the subsequent common foods: refined white bread, polished white rice, processed white pasta, peeled potatoes, commercially-produced corn flakes, indulgent ice cream, crispy rice cereals, cooked carrots, and sweeteners (with the exception of fructose).

The gastrointestinal (GI) tract can prove to be highly beneficial in the formulation of your dietary regimen. For instance, it is advisable to consume foods classified as high GI promptly following a rigorous exercise session in order to amplify the insulin response and effectively replenish muscle glycogen reserves. Consuming foods that fall within the low glycemic index (GI) range can facilitate weight loss, therefore it is advisable to prioritize the consumption of such foods, while restricting the intake of high GI foods during the course of the day. The following chart presents a selection of frequently consumed food items:

The following fruits and vegetables have a low glycemic index (less than 55): apple, broccoli, cherries, grapefruit, orange, pear, and tomatoes.

Foods with a glycemic index between 56 and 69 include banana, brown rice, oatmeal, popcorn, sweet potato, white rice, and whole wheat bread.

Foods with a high glycemic index (70 and above) include bagels, doughnuts, rice cakes, pretzels, watermelons, white bread, and white potatoes.

It is apparent that your current diet comprises all the food items listed in the aforementioned category. Rest assured, the current state of affairs shall soon undergo transformation. Upon completing this literary work, you will have successfully altered your dietary proclivities and embarked upon the path to acquiring a slender and muscular physique.

Counting Carbohydrates

For individuals embarking on an active lifestyle and seeking to shed pounds, it is recommended to limit daily carbohydrate consumption to a range of 100 to 150 grams. The main sources of carbohydrates ought to consist predominantly of vegetables and fruits. Additionally, it is possible to consume modest portions of nutritious starches, such as sweet potatoes and potatoes (with the peel intact), in conjunction with whole grains such as brown rice and oats.

There is a pervasive curiosity among individuals regarding the healthiness of fruits, owing to their inherent sweetness and potential contribution to adipose tissue accumulation in the body. Indeed, fruits do contain fructose, a compound of greater chemical complexity compared to sucrose, which is found in sugar. Therefore, in the event that your body is subjected to both substances, it will require greater physiological exertion to metabolize the former in comparison to the latter. In the course of this process, it ultimately facilitates the combustion of a greater amount of adipose tissue. Therefore, it is incorrect to believe that consuming fruit has negative health implications, unless one indulges in excessively sugary fruits on a continuous basis. Nevertheless, it may be necessary to exercise caution if you possess elevated sugar levels within your physiological system.

To enhance and expedite weight loss, it is essential to restrict daily carbohydrate consumption within the range of 50 to 100 grams. This range is equally suitable for individuals with Celiac disease or any other condition characterized by carbohydrate sensitivity. Place your focus on consuming mainly vegetables and restricting the intake of fruit to one to three servings per day, while minimizing the consumption of starchy carbohydrates.

In order to significantly enhance your metabolic rate, it is recommended to consume a daily range of 20 to 50 grams of carbohydrates. Consuming fewer than 50 grams per day will induce a metabolic state called ketosis, wherein the body begins to utilize its fat reserves as a source of energy. You should only eat low GI carbohydrate vegetables, such as leafy greens, and trace carbohydrates from raw nuts, seeds, avocados, and berries. I advise you to exercise caution by seeking counsel from a medical professional prior to implementing any substantial modifications to your dietary regimen, in order to preempt any potential health complications that may arise.

Developing muscular strength and size within a 30-day timeframe

Perhaps you are questioning the feasibility of such a prospect. It is possible to achieve significant reduction in body fat over a period of 30 days without engaging in exhaustive exercise routines, should one so desire. It is feasible provided that one diligently adheres to the guidelines of their meal plan and acknowledges that the concise 30-day duration allows little leeway for laxity.

Now, what is the level of possibility for this? There are several fundamental measures that can be implemented to optimize outcomes while minimizing muscle wastage. We highly recommend that you experiment with the recommendations provided herein over the span of one month, as the positive impact on your physique will become apparent in due course.

1. Optimize your training duration.

To optimize caloric expenditure within the confines of a single strength training session, it is imperative to capitalize on every minute spent in the gym. Please direct your attention towards incorporating various types of compound exercises that engage multiple muscle groups and joints. Participate in physical activities such as bench presses, push-ups, rows, and squats. These exercises effectively focus on the major muscle groups and guarantee a substantial impact on fat combustion.

## 2. Scale back cardio

Devoting an excessive amount of time to treadmill workouts can yield significantly detrimental consequences. Excessive cardio training combined with a caloric deficit can lead to a state of overtraining. The human body necessitates energy and shall demonstrate resistance in the event of inadequate recuperation. This phenomenon has the potential to exert a substantial influence on your body from a hormonal standpoint, resulting in various effects such as diminished testosterone production, accelerated muscle catabolism, and elevated cortisol secretion.

## 3. Fuel up properly

It is advised to consume a pre-workout meal approximately thirty minutes prior to commencing a training session. Select an option consisting of a combination of rapidly and slowly digestible carbohydrates, such as a serving of oatmeal accompanied by a portion of fruit. Nevertheless, following physical activity, one has the option of consuming a combination of carbohydrates, protein, and nutritious fats, such as eggs, whole-grain toast, and a modest portion of turkey from free-range sources. It is important to maintain regular meal times and avoid prolonged periods without eating. Choosing to forego meals leads to the depletion of carbohydrates, followed by lipid stores, and eventually results in muscle catabolism. Drastically reducing caloric intake can result in the degradation of muscle tissue. Consuming three meals daily that are high in protein content will sufficiently provide the anabolic stimulus necessary for your muscles to enhance their strength.

4. Sleep more

Optimal restorative sleep enhances both cognitive function and physical vitality. The insufficient acquisition of restorative sleep frequently results in depleted levels of energy, compromised ability to concentrate, increased body weight, along with an elevated susceptibility to depression, diabetes, hypertension, and obesity.

Rest intervals and rejuvenation are critical.

In addition to ensuring proper nutrition, inadequate rest can have the detrimental effect of reversing the anabolic process and inducing a catabolic state, which is harmful to the body. The impact of the diet on muscle hypertrophy is determined by the interaction between protein metabolism and meals consumed within the time frame of 24-48 hours following a resistance exercise session. It is important to be aware that there exists a specific threshold for muscle growth determined by factors such as age, gender, and genetics. Males possess a higher level of testosterone in comparison to females, consequently facilitating the development of larger and stronger muscular structures.

Once you have completed your training, it is crucial to engage in a gradual cool-down period for a few minutes in order to maintain proper circulation. The expeditious deceleration of one's body results in a reduced rate of clearance of lactate and acid, consequently leading to the process of regeneration. Furthermore, it is imperative to engage in a comprehensive stretching regimen to effectively eliminate metabolic waste from intensified muscular structures, while also facilitating enhanced cellular receptivity to a wider range of nutrients. Hence, it is imperative that you partake in stretching and gentle exercises during days when you are not engaged in regular training sessions.

Gentle, effortless motions, along with stretching and application of heat, facilitate the enhanced flow of blood, thus promoting the exchange of nutrients and oxygen within the muscle cells. Experiment with the utilization of saunas and hot baths, along with engaging in moderate jogging and leisurely strolls. Nonetheless, exercise caution to avoid exerting excessive strain on your muscles. Restrict your movements within a range that you are accustomed to.

It is imperative to prioritize adequate hydration following training, as all physiological processes within the body occur in the aqueous milieu. When one experiences dehydration, the normal functions of digestion, restructuring, and transportation of nutrients are all adversely impacted. In the context of long-term outcomes, the significance of endurance training cannot be overstated, as it effectively enhances multiple physiological systems and the overall integrity of the organism that are indispensable in facilitating the recuperative process.

## Prominent Errors Hampering Your Muscle Development

Bodybuilding necessitates adherence to discipline as opposed to indulgence in excess. In pursuit of greater muscular development, we may inadvertently become a hindrance to our own progress. Bodybuilders often tend to make certain errors that can be attributed to the inclination of going above and beyond what is necessary, when in fact a more conservative approach would have yielded superior results. By refraining from making these errors, you can prevent the unnecessary expenditure of your time, finances, and efforts.

## Consuming an excessive amount of dietary supplements

Dietary supplements are designed to bridge the nutritional deficiencies inherent in your overall food intake, contributing to enhanced outcomes derived from your physical exercise endeavors. They do not, nor will they ever, serve as a replacement for a balanced diet or diligent effort.

Certain individuals have a propensity to exhaust a significant portion of their monthly allocation for sustenance on excessively marketed dietary supplements, overlooking the fact that what they truly require are fundamental whole food items such as steak, sweet potatoes, and other essential sources. These dietary necessities can be adequately complemented by basic elements including protein, creatine, fish oil, and pre-workout supplements.

In essence, attaining proficiency in vital nutrition would yield superior outcomes compared to relying on exceptional supplementation while maintaining a substandard diet.

Incorporating additional training sessions and exercises.

Many individuals dedicate a significant amount of their time engaged in online discussions, deliberating upon the existence or non-existence of overtraining. The phenomenon of excessive training is present and can pose hazardous implications on one's physical well-being.

The prevalent mindset of "more is better" in bodybuilding should be cautioned against, particularly when it pertains to the duration and frequency of exercise sessions. This is because muscle growth actually occurs outside of the gym, following the completion of workouts.

If one engages in vigorous training, it is possible that the physical exertion exerted in the gym might result in micro-tears and muscular trauma. It is the physical activity conducted beyond the confines of the fitness facility that contributes to the repair of this physiological damage; this includes nutritive intake, hydration, mobility exercises, dietary supplements, and notably, quality sleep. Nevertheless, should you persist in subjecting a muscle to intense training prior to the completion of its repair period, you not only deprive yourself of further development but also expose yourself to increased risk of injury and unnecessary discomfort.

In order to facilitate the growth and strengthening of your muscles, it is necessary to prioritize ample recovery rather than limiting it. It is imperative to ensure that your muscles are afforded sufficient time to fully recuperate prior to engaging them in further training sessions. By doing so, you will experience accelerated gains without the risk of sustaining any injuries.

# WAYS TO GROW MUSCLE

Building body muscle? Subsequently, one must possess a level of fervor in order to initiate the task at hand. There are occasions when going to the gym may appear burdensome, however, by faithfully following a purposeful exercise routine, we move closer to our intended goal and reap the associated advantages. Engaging in an intermittent training routine would result in repetitive revisiting of previous material, whereby the initial phase of any training program, following the warm-up, would primarily involve restoring muscle tone as opposed to building upon it. If you are able to motivate yourself to engage fully and exert maximum effort, a significant portion of the challenge has already been overcome. However, it is important not to become excessively engrossed. Seek to find appropriate and suitable inspiration without exceeding the necessary limit.

Additionally, it is crucial to bear in mind that unchecked enthusiasm can bring about negative consequences. Devoting time to the gym is essential for achieving physical fitness. However, it is equally valid to acknowledge that excessive time spent in the gym or attempting to cram an excessive amount of exercise within that time can be counterproductive. Consequently, this will lead to self-infliction of harm, or at the very least, significantly complicate the process of maintaining a consistent routine. It is crucial to possess a certain degree of adaptability, as an excessive development of muscle can potentially impede one's flexibility.

The proposed solution entails developing a structured routine that incorporates designated periods of relaxation. By achieving this, you will establish a practical framework for yourself, yielding tangible outcomes that can be monitored and analyzed for educational purposes. Do not haste in the process of developing muscle mass. Things take time. If the task is expedited, the potential consequences could include injuries and illnesses. To enhance one's certainty, it is advisable to seek guidance from individuals who have achieved notable success in the field of bodybuilding.